Securing Serenity

Securing Serenity

SURVIVING A LOVED ONE'S ADDICTION

Larissa Theison, LCSW

ISBN: 0692684476
ISBN 13: 9780692684474

Table of Contents

CHAPTER 1

An Introduction: Training for Survival

This survivor's guide is designed to be a supportive tool for anyone who has a loved one struggling with addiction. It is intended to be a no-nonsense approach to learning how to cope with the addiction and create lasting, genuine change within yourself in order to (re)discover your zest for life and take action to support your loved one's steps toward recovery.

It is exceedingly hard to live with addiction—not only because it is difficult to understand how the disease works but also because of the total chaos it creates in the lives of the people who love the addict. Addiction is unsettling because it has enormous power over the people it touches. It's important to know that you are not alone. Many stories you hear about addiction touch you closely because, unfortunately, the track of the illness is always very similar. But your story is yours to tell, and no one knows exactly what you have been through, except for you. Because of this, you are the expert in your own healing, and this workbook is designed to be a key to unlocking the wisdom and tools you already have within you.

This workbook will assist with learning to manage the impacts of addiction in your life, while giving you the freedom to navigate and process through how it has affected you. It is *never* only the addict who is suffering from the disease caused by drug or alcohol abuse; you have experienced misery yourself and have been trying to manage it as best as you can.

As you go through this workbook, always have a pen and journal handy to take notes as you read and complete the "Daily Meditations" and "Survival Step" tasks. This workbook will be most helpful if you work through it in order, as it has been designed sequentially to assist first with understanding and then with healing. Don't do the tasks halfheartedly, as you will cheat yourself of the lasting benefits of truly working through the issues at hand. If at any time you are struck by some thought or revelation and it is not one of the tasks in the book, then by all means, take some time to work through it in your journal. The "Daily Meditations" are words from other knowledgeable teachers and spiritual leaders whose wisdom have aided in my own journey of healing.

If you are reading this, it is likely that you have spent so much time trying to take care of your loved one that you have neglected yourself along the way. Don't shortchange yourself through this workbook by not giving the assignments and tasks your 100 percent. Don't do it all at once; do one, *maybe* two sections at a time—it is important to sit with the material after you have completed it to allow it to saturate your spirit. Also, do not hesitate to reach out for other help in the community, be it through Al-Anon meetings, other therapy, or spiritual counseling. This workbook is designed to be a tool on the journey toward healing, but it is **not** a substitute for other support in the community. It is important to have many resources that you can utilize to ensure your success and well-being.

Loving someone who is an addict leaves people feeling overwhelmed, powerless, uncertain, and stressed. Give yourself and your loved one the greatest gift of all—learn to take care of *yourself* through the crisis of the addiction. Cure *yourself* of the continuous disease that plagues you so many of your waking moments.

Please note—any events, names, details, and identifying information in the stories throughout have been altered to protect confidentiality. Also, because this condition impacts anyone of any gender, the gender pronouns "him/himself" and "her/herself" are used interchangeably throughout the book.

If you are ready to begin this journey, move forward with the work ahead and flourish. Best wishes on the incredible journey of securing serenity for your soul.

Sincerely,
Larissa Theison

CHAPTER 2

Dis-Ease of a Soul: Inside Addiction, What You *Have* to Know

<u>Meditation for Today:</u> I am beginning a journey of releasing the hold addiction has had over my life. When we can no longer change the things happening around us, then we have to consider what has to change for us. What are the parts of my life I want to change? Settle in, and take a moment to allow answers to rise within you.

An addiction is a disease, and when it strikes a person, he or she will have no power to control it. It's difficult to grasp the idea of addiction as a disease, but it is important to consider the concept of a medical disease to begin to understand.

If you think about a person who has cancer, a medically diagnosed disease, what characteristics come to mind that make cancer a disease? Jot down a few ideas below:

1. ____
2. ____
3. ____
4. ____
5. ____

You have probably identified some of the following: Cancer is an illness with *genetic factors* that spreads over time; it gets *progressively worse without treatment*; it weakens the individual by *attacking the body, mind, and spirit*; it *cannot be cured* (only managed and may go into remission); and if untreated, it will lead to *destruction of the body and mind, and subsequent death*. So, you guessed it—addiction defined as a disease is the same. You can look at the characteristics of a medically diagnosed disease and see that addiction wreaks havoc in a similar way. In this workbook, this condition will be referenced as "dis-ease" in order to capture the scientific characteristics along with the psychological and emotional impacts. Addiction creates dis-ease among all of those it touches. It not only affects the physical and mental health of the addict but also generates significant emotional strain and stress for the user and the people who love him—hence dis-ease.

Like all people living with a loved one with an addiction, you struggle to understand why the dis-ease has so much power over the person you know and love. It's as though the addiction is driving the airplane, and your loved one isn't even a copilot. It may seem more like he or she is stuck in the cargo hold with little say over where the plane goes. This, in part, explains why the person behaves in ways that are totally uncharacteristic of the person you know is hiding inside of the addiction. Oftentimes, persons struggling with addiction express feeling completely out of control of the actions they take when using. They may feel compelled by a force that is extraordinarily stronger than their will or their ability to resist. I have heard addicts describe that when they are in the throes of the addiction, using is like breathing—it is essential to living and getting through each moment of the day. So it makes sense how difficult it can be to break its hold on your loved one.

However, addiction being a disease does not excuse accountability for actions and choices that are made. Just as someone with cancer can choose to change his or her whole lifestyle for healthier alternatives and seek treatment, so can an addict. Oftentimes, though, they will not seek the help needed until life gets to a point of being completely dis-eased in all areas. Life becomes so out of control and miserable that there is no other alternative besides changing. They often have to hit rock bottom to start building their lives back up. They get sick and tired of being sick and tired, and often it is only then they may begin moving toward recovery. Your choices in your relationship with the addict, yourself, and your family can support your loved one in moving closer to recovery or deeper into the dis-ease. We'll explore this more in later sections, but first, complete this Survival Step.

Survival Step: How have you seen the person you love change as the addiction has progressed? How has this affected you and your family?

____

____

____

____

____

____

____

CHAPTER 3

Enabling Eliminated: How You Stop Supporting the Dis-ease

__Meditation for Today:__ Addiction is like an ocean that is ebbing and flowing, no obvious end in sight. It has many intricate parts that are complex and difficult to understand. Allow yourself to settle in and consider the image of floating along, accepting the ebb and flow of the waves as a force that is wholly beyond your control. Now consider the ways you can be empowered to change your own situation as you are in the ebb and flow of the ocean's waves.

People throw around the words "enabling" and "codependence" a lot when describing the family members of addicts. If you are living with an addict in your life, it is likely that you receive these words with twinges of guilt and worry and wonder if you are one of these "enabling codependents." This survivor's guide is here to say first, no matter what you've done or where you are in this process, *you have done the best you can with where you are and what you have.*

Andi has lived with her mom's alcoholism her whole life. As a result, she essentially raised herself and has had to watch her mom make some really dangerous decisions. It is not uncommon for her mom to be arrested for fighting people and getting behind the wheel of the car while intoxicated. On many of these occasions, Andi has been in the car screaming, crying, and begging her mom, "Please, Mom, stop! I'm scared!" Andi knew her mom was in there somewhere, but when she was drinking, she became meaner, angrier, and did things she never did when she was sober. Some days while her mom slept off the effects of the previous night, Andi would go around their house and dump out all of the alcohol she could find. When her mom woke up, she would become enraged and beat Andi before she went up the street to get more whiskey.

Other days, Andi just wanted her mom to be happy, so she would give her the money she had earned from her babysitting job. Money she knew her mom would use to buy alcohol and cigarettes. Andi felt helpless and scared a great deal of the time, and she worried that every time her mother left the house it would be the last time she ever saw her alive. She felt ravaged with guilt and uncertainty because nothing she ever did made her mom quit drinking.

She talked to her best friend about her greatest fear—being called in to identify her mom's body and never having the chance to have the relationship she knew they could have.

Just as it is true with Andi, there is absolutely no judgment for any of the decisions <u>you</u> have made while managing the effects of addiction on your life! In fact, it is safe to say there are no mistakes because you have been learning to adjust to the impacts in your life and have been doing the best you can to manage. Even when Andi was buying her mom's alcohol, she was trying to navigate an uncertain path to find even moments of happiness and joy. Over time, she discovered that this wasn't something that helped her or her mom in the long run, and she was able to make some changes that felt right for her. Unfortunately, there is no exact guide that says "do this" and "don't do that." To most, it would probably make sense that Andi needed to stop spending her money on her mom's addiction, but when that was the only smile she saw from her mom that month, it was a difficult decision to make. Over time, Andi did see that this was not bringing genuine happiness or content-ment to her or her mom and led only to feelings of resentment and bitterness towards her mom. She knew she needed to make changes that would truly support any recovery steps taken by her mom, and this meant never spending a dime on her mom's alcoholism again.

Survival Step: Write yourself a letter—include only praise for how you have managed the hardship of the addiction, with the intention of comforting yourself. Remember: no negative judgments allowed!

Survival Step: Now that you have written the letter, go back through and read it aloud to yourself. This may feel very strange, but it *so* important not to skip this step! If you have written any "you should haves," "I wish you would haves," or "too bad you didn'ts"—then go back through and change those statements to be affirming and supportive. Take out or change anything in the letter that is guilt-inducing. Remember, what's the past is past; you are in the *here and now*, learning a new set of skills to move forward.

With this workbook and any other support you can find, you will discover a number of strategies that can help with not supporting the dis-ease any longer. In Andi's treatment, it was important that she find answers within herself to help her to know what she needed in her own life. One very important piece of this was breaking the cycle of addiction that ran rampant in her family. She also had to work on her grief and loss associated with her and her mom not getting to have the relationship she had always dreamed of having. She made some hard decisions about where it was safe to live and ended up moving out of her mom's and into her aunt's house to finish school. Her mom still abuses alcohol, and it is still hard for Andi to see the devastation in her mom's life. However, Andi decided it was best for her to love her mom from a distance and continue the work of building a successful life for herself.

Andi will never let go of the hope that her mom will enter into recovery, but in the meantime, she resolved that she won't let alcohol control another day of her own life. Not everyone makes the same decisions as Andi, and you may not either. It is most important to explore what will lead you to securing your serenity, even if the storm continues to rage in your loved one's life.

If you are operating out of guilt, you cannot be effective in dealing with the addiction. Remember Dr. Sparks Lunney's three Cs related to family members coping with addiction: you didn't *cause* it, you can't *cure* it, and you can't *control* it. This the foundation for understanding that you absolutely do not bear responsibility for the addiction, and you cannot control whether or not the addict changes her life. If someone you love is self-destructing, it's the most natural thing in the world to want to do something to change that; to try to save her. Andi struggled desperately with going back and forth between supporting her mom's drinking and trying to erase it from their lives. Unfortunately, just like with any other disease, only time and the person's response to it will determine if her life will change for the better. You can certainly be one of the factors in your loved one's life pushing toward recovery and wellness, but you cannot *make* the person with the addiction change.

Survival Step: Get a small piece of paper, or a Post-it note, and write down the mantra: "I didn't cause it, I can't cure it, and I can't control it." Post this somewhere where you will see it often for a daily reminder.

The only power of influence you have on the addiction is how you respond to it. Your choices can also be one element of the addict's journey that will help push her in the direction of recovery and wellness. So let's explore what people mean when they talk about enabling and codependence:

"To enable," by definition, is "to allow." To enable the addiction is to act (or not act) in ways that support the substance abuse. Sometimes enabling can be overt actions taken by an individual to protect the addict. Andi would sometimes find herself offering to pay for her mom's alcohol to make her happy and keep the peace. Other common examples may be calling in to work for your husband and telling the boss that he doesn't feel well; or paying your son's car payment and buying him groceries because he spent his money on drugs; or bailing him out of jail after the most recent arrest for disorderly conduct or driving under the influence. Other times, enabling can be actions *not* taken, such as ignoring the elephant in the room, not speaking openly with the person about the impacts of her addiction, or not setting limits for yourself and the other person.

"Codependence," in a nutshell, is when helping someone hurts you, or when you are only okay when someone else is okay. This would include any action you take to try to "cure" or "take care of" the addict but doing so brings harm or pain into your own life. This can mean you take on consequences that are meant for the addict in order to prevent her from experiencing all of the pain of it. Or it can simply be emotional distress from obsessing about how to help or only feeling like you can be emotionally okay when the people you love are okay. Andi would cut classes to make sure her mom made it to her job. If she wasn't there to wake her up, her mom would often oversleep and lose her job. But then Andi's grades and good standing in school began to plummet. Other examples may be bailing your daughter out of jail and being unable to afford to do other things you needed to do. Or maybe you spend too much time worrying about how to help, and you cannot focus at your job and are losing sleep at night. You may chase your partner around, trying to control and monitor every move and behavior, giving all of your time and thoughts to your worry about what he is doing—and when you have spent all your time and energy but your partner is still using, you feel resentful, empty, ineffective, and alone. You, in turn, find yourself suffering as a result of the addiction.

It's important to figure out how your own behavior may be contributing to the addiction so you can stop it and move toward supporting recovery behaviors. But remember the piece about not judging yourself for the past? It is critically important to be aware of this at all times, or you may wind up beating yourself up over so-called "mistakes." The only use for "guilt" in this moment is identifying when you have felt it so you can pinpoint times that you have enabled the person you love. Ultimately, your focus must be on noticing these situations and determining *proactive* ways to act upon your insights in order to put your energy and support into recovery work. Then, praise yourself for your wisdom and go to work developing your skill set.

Survival Step: In what ways have you felt the guilt of enabling the addiction? What things have you done or not done to support the addiction?

____

____

____

____

Survival Step: What have you done in an attempt to help the addict that has hurt you, physically, emotionally, or spiritually? How have you allowed the dis-ease to begin to control your life? (Remember, this can even be a pattern of thinking or obsessing about your loved one)

____

____

____

____

Survival Step: What kind of life will _you_ be living if you continue with the status quo?

____

____

____

____

Survival Step: Write a letter to the loved one telling him or her what you are going to be doing to change yourself so that you can support steps taken toward your own well-being and recovery. Explain how you will stop investing yourself in the dis-ease.

____

____

____

____

CHAPTER 4

Dealing with the Damage: Identifying How the Dis-ease Affects You

__Meditation for Today:__ Take a moment to settle into this moment and try to think of a one-word answer to each of these questions: What do you want to release related to the addiction's hold over your life? What do you want to bring more of to this situation? When you find the words, take a moment and pair them with your breathing—on the exhale, pair it with the word of what you want to release; on the inhale, pair it the word of the quality you want to bring more of to this situation.

Addiction takes an enormously painful toll on family members and loved ones while it wreaks havoc in the user's life. You will need to determine what has changed for you in order to take proactive steps to heal. In this section, you will identify the changes in yourself and, in the next, you will do more intensive work on healing the wounds.

Survival Step: How has your life changed in response to the anxiety/worry about the addiction?

- Physically, what's different? (Think about your physical energy and if your body/health has changed.)

____

____

____

____

____

- Emotionally, how do you feel most of the time?

____

____

____

____

- Mentally, what consumes your thoughts?

____

____

____

____

- Spiritually, how have you changed?

____

____

____

____

Time for a Survival Self-Inventory!

Exercise: Yes   No

1. I hardly ever have the time to work out.   ____   ____
2. I never have the energy it takes to get active.   ____   ____
3. I avoid/put off following an exercise schedule.   ____   ____
4. I can name ways that I could get more active.   ____   ____

What do you need to change about your exercise habits so that they fit your lifestyle? What priority shifts will have to occur?

____

____

____

____

Eating Habits: Yes   No

5. I eat a lot of fast food and junk foods.   ____   ____
6. I know what needs to change about my eating habits.   ____   ____
7. I eat three to six balanced meals per day.   ____   ____
8. I eat plenty of fruits and vegetables.   ____   ____

What do you need to change about your eating habits, and what are some simple steps to doing it?

____

____

____

____

Sleeping Habits: Yes   No

  9. I sleep seven to nine hours every night.   ____   ____
10. I feel well rested throughout most of the day.   ____   ____
11. When I try to sleep, worried thoughts race in my mind.   ____   ____
12. I frequently oversleep or sleep late.   ____   ____
13. I drink a lot of caffeine.   ____   ____

Lastly, what needs to change about your sleeping habits, and what are some simple steps that may help you get more rest?

____

____

____

____

____

Some tips on the healthy lifestyle inventories: Priorities will need to change, especially if you are going to eat healthier, exercise more, and sleep better. But the benefits will be well worth the investment if you can find a way to make even some simple changes.

Possible ideas for increasing physical activity: Buy an exercise video, get up thirty to forty-five minutes earlier, and start your day with physical activity. Park farther away when you go shopping or to work so you have to increase the number of steps you take each day. Take the stairs anytime you can. You must prioritize physical activity to ensure you will follow through on any new plans, even small ones. We will always find a way to make time for things that are important to us.

For improved eating habits, eat something for breakfast every day. Make sure you stock your kitchen with healthy snacks, whole wheat/grain bread, plenty of fruits and vegetables, and make your lunch every day. Then, have the healthy staples in the kitchen at all times and try to avoid having ready access to unhealthy food in your home. As much as possible, especially as you are starting new habits, try for fast preparation foods to make it easier to change some of your eating habits. Make lists and follow them when you shop for groceries, and go to the store when you are full—if you don't buy it at the grocery store, you won't have to resist it at home when you feel tempted.

For sleep, first try some winding-down activities and relaxation or deep breathing a few minutes before you go to bed. There are many free apps for your smartphone with guided relaxation and mindfulness activities to improve sleep. If you continue to struggle to get a good night's sleep, consider seeing a therapist or other support in order to have an outlet for your worry, fears, hurt, or anxiety. You may also want to contact your doctor for other options. We all feel 100 percent better when we are getting enough sleep. If we don't, our energy is low and emotions run high and sensitive. Take charge of your emotions by taking these few small steps. They will yield enormous results.

Remember, you are worthy of the investment in your own personal well-being. You may have been spending a lot of your time and energy worrying about your loved one. While your dedication and commitment to your family is important, taking care of yourself will be so valuable in helping you find peace, wisdom, and a sense of well-being. It is important that you put just as much energy and work into yourself as you do for anyone you love. In fact, we can't fully be present and love others until we are doing the same for ourselves. If you start by loving and caring for yourself, you will find strength and endurance for the journey ahead.

CHAPTER 5

Coping with the Chaos: Healing the Wounds of Addiction

__Meditation for Today:__ Hope is the antidote to despair. It's the piece of peace you can find within yourself when it seems like the addiction will never end. Take a moment and consider what gives you hope in this moment? For the next month? Year? Allow yourself to float on the hope for a few moments, and then try to carry it with you through the day.

You have likely been through so much pain and strife because of ceaseless worry and fear for the person you love. Take, for example, Sandy, a mother who lost her four children to the state due to problems that are related to her drug addiction. In her moments of sobriety, she insists that she would never have abused her children had she not been in a meth haze, not thinking clearly and seeing her children as one more obstacle to the next high. In the moments in which she gets off the drugs and into treatment, she finds that she missed out on so much of her children's lives. The reality of all she has missed and all she has to do to get them back seems too overwhelming to consider. Plus, she knows that she has tried so many times to stop using and has never been able to manage more than a few weeks of sobriety. Sandy knows she struggles to take care of herself and is afraid of how she will affect her kids' lives if she relapses again. In her mind, it's not a matter of "if" but "when" she relapses again. This, coupled with the shame and guilt over what she did when she was using, makes her wonder if her kids are better off without her. Allowing the state to take her children away so that someone else will have a chance to parent them seems like a better idea than having to go through what it would take to recover all that lost time and make up for past mistakes.

While grappling with the enormity of all of these questions, Sandy finds herself checking herself out of the most recent inpatient treatment admission against the advice of the people who are trying to convince her that she has a life worth living and reasons to continue trying to stay sober. Leaving treatment was not so much about being able to use again as it was symbolizing the final acceptance that her children would be better off without her in their lives. Sandy finds herself back in the world of drug use and all the dangerous activities and relationships that go with it, and her children are left wondering, "Why did mommy choose meth over me?" These questions are impossible to answer. More significantly, it is often not the right question to be asking about an addict who says she needs the drug like her next breath. Or some-one whose self-worth is so non-existent that she believes that ultimately, her children will be better off without her and her mistakes. Anyone grappling with the questions about what keeps the addict going back to the substances and why the family's love wasn't enough to cure him/her needs support with gaining more understanding of addiction. Sandy's children stand the best chance of not repeating their mom's mistakes and keeping drugs or alcohol from destroying their own lives if they get a lot of support early. "Why did my loved one choose meth over me?" is an example of one of the many questions that, left unsettled and unresolved, can bring continued emotional wreckage to all of our lives.

At times, it seems so hopeless that anything will change, and it is easy to get sucked into the despair of ques-tioning why all of this has happened. You feel powerless to make any changes and aren't sure what is the right thing to do. This survivor's guide is here to say that the best thing you can do for yourself and your loved one is to begin to heal yourself—today—right now. Your loved one may not be at a point where he can heal himself; but you are reading this now, so you are ready to begin the journey to mend your soul.

Survival Step: You will experience many mixed emotions while witnessing the destruction of the addiction. Write down some of the feelings you have had in reaction to the addiction—and make sure you focus on feel-ings, not thoughts.

____

____

____

____

____

Take a look at what you have written. Circle any that you feel guilty for feeling. Why do you feel this way? How much more painful is it to feel the guilt on top of the anger, resentment, sadness, etc.? Nothing you feel is ever wrong, unfounded, undeserved, or unfair. How you deal with the feelings *from here on* will make all the differ-ence because the hard truth is that you will feel all of these again if the person does not quit using. If you cannot validate your own feelings and learn to cope with them, you will continue in destructive patterns of your own.

Survival Step: Look at your list of feelings again—pick the top three or four that you feel most often, or with the most intensity, and underline them. Write a letter to the addict expressing these feelings and explain why you feel them. This is not a letter you will give to the person, so use it to vent all of your thoughts and feelings.

____

____

Survival Step: Now add (either at the end of the letter, or in a PS) all about how much you love him or her and all of your hopes for the person.

Survival Step: Read the letter aloud as though you are reading it to the person—and then be content with sending the thoughts into the world. You may want to tear up or burn the letter in order to represent your own process of letting go of the responsibility of trying to control or change the addict's behavior. Write any additional reflections in the space provided below:

____

____

____

____

____

____

____

____

____

____

It is important to hold onto hope that the addict will recover, and since thoughts have energy, it is important to send that hope out into the world often. However, don't confuse hope with intent to change the addict. Hope is an instrument of comfort that must be nurtured because it means you are not living in despair. Attempting to change the addict only takes you back into the vicious cycle of trying to control something over which you have absolutely no power.

CHAPTER 6

Take Your Life Back: Steps Toward Reparation and Moving On

**Meditation for Today:** It is okay to be kind to myself. I am worthy of the care and nurturing that my body, soul, and spirit need. It is okay to be kind to myself.

As you are moving forward in your own journey of healing from the wounds of the addiction, consider the life you have always wanted. You may have hopes of getting your life back to the way it was before addiction was in the picture. It's hard for John and Jamie, parents who have been struggling for years with their daughter, Samantha's, heroin addiction. They feel as if they have tried everything to help her but nothing has worked longer than a few weeks at a time. Looking back, they see that it started with Samantha feeling bullied and having more problems in school, resulting in hanging out with the wrong crowd. She entered into a downward spiral that ended up with their daughter running away from home and getting hooked on heroin. As parents, Jamie and John are desperate for answers so they can get their daughter back before it is too late, but she says she has no intention of quitting anytime soon.

Her parents continue to question and obsess over what they could have done differently and where they went wrong. They struggle every day with feeling like failures who don't deserve to move on with their lives. How can parents find any semblance of happiness or joy when their daughter is on a slow path of self-destruction? They love their daughter and only want good things for her, but it has become more and more clear to them that they cannot _force_ her to make the changes to improve her life. They need to learn what they can about their daughter's devastating illness and determine what is right for them to do—for themselves, their relationship, the rest of their family, and their daughter.

When we get clear with our own values and goals and act in line with what will help us to recover from the effects of addiction on our own lives, we can discover more peace and serenity about our role in recovery. As John and Jamie started doing the right things for themselves, they saw that they were clearer and more united in responding to their daughter when she needed their support. The pain did not evaporate, but they became more empowered to help other families while continuing to support recovery behaviors for themselves and their daughter.

It is important that you start figuring out how you want to live your life. Yours is truly the only life you will ever be able to live. As much as you may desire change for your loved one, yours is the only destiny that you can change. Yes, you will be instrumental in the lives of so many you touch, but the question comes back to how you want to *be* in your own and others' lives. As you live more in line with your wisdom and serenity, you will become a powerful instrument of change and hope, even for others who are suffering the way you have.

Survival Step: Let's consider this. Get into a comfortable seated position, somewhere quiet, and ask yourself, "What kind of life do I desire?" Ponder this question for several moments and allow yourself to uncover the many layers that may exist within the answer. As you uncover one answer, allow that to lead you to your next. When your mind interjects any negative beliefs that doubt or question your abilities to achieve this life, notice those thoughts and move forward. Notice the negative beliefs but try to filter through them so you don't allow the self-defeating thoughts to clutter up your vision for yourself.

After you have pondered the question, complete the following:

1. Jot down your ideas below for the kind of life you want to have. (And remember, don't limit yourself because of what is or isn't realistic!)

2. Jot down some of the negative or doubting thoughts that entered into your mind as you thought about living this life.

____

____

____

3. Create a Transformation Statement that captures what you want in your life. Use the format below, or choose one of your own:

    "Today I choose [insert word(s) related to #1], and I give myself permission to live my life with joy and abundance. I commit to living my life free of [insert words from #2 that you are trying to leave behind] and filling that space with loving kindness for my soul."

    ____

    ____

    ____

    ____

    ____

4. Now, use the next blank page for the following instructions. At the top, write your Transformation Statement. Now, get some old magazines or pictures online, and select different pictures or words that represent anything you want to pursue or achieve; anything in line with your answer to #1. Use this as a compass: a reminder that each moment—each breath—is one more opportunity to live abundantly. Dream big, and go for it!

Transformation Statement:

CHAPTER 7

Rediscovering Your Identity: Freedom from Addiction

__Meditation for Today:__ Reconsider that part of yourself that wants to live a life of joy and freedom. In this work so far, we have spent time considering how pain and suffering go hand-in-hand when there is not acceptance, or a release of what you are unable to change. For at least three cycles of deep breaths, take a moment and inhale "freedom" and exhale "surrender."

t's time to rediscover yourself—you remember, the person buried deep inside of you, the one who existed before the addiction took over so much of your life? It happens to many family members of addicts at one time or another; the worry becomes such a burden and consumes your thoughts so much that it nearly becomes your life. Well, it's time to start uncovering the passionate parts of yourself so that you can move toward your wellness, peace, and serenity—and find yourself in the process.

Survival Step: Let's take another self-inventory. This one's a little different and is going to take some thought/writing.

1. What are the things/people/ideas/activities you:
    a. Like?

    ____

    ____

    b. Love?

    ____

    ____

c. Dislike?

____

____

2. What are the things you know to be true about yourself? (Examples: "I'm a great cook, I enjoy gardening, I love to travel…")

____

____

____

____

3. If money and time were not a factor, what would you do with your life? You can use your Transformation Statement for some of the ideas, but also remember to include the seemingly small activities you may not have thought to include. In other words, the list could not only include something grandiose, such as backpacking for six months across Australia, but also humbler pastimes such as taking an art class or reading a romance novel.

____

____

____

____

4. What are some things you would like to learn?

____

____

5. Now—pick *at least one* of the activities you listed in exercises three and four—and go do it! Put it on a calendar, call up that old friend, and set a time to get together. Take some time to make some calls and do online research about things you want to learn to do, or find fun activities in your community. The sky is the limit, but make sure you are setting some real and achievable goals. It doesn't have to cost a lot of money or time. Just find ways to make time for the basics of truly experiencing a full and enriched life. If you would like to take an art class, many community centers offer them free or for low cost. If you add one new thing per month to your calendar, you would be starting something amazing for yourself. Then, after you have done these activities a time or two, write about what it was like to be able to free yourself to *choose* how you spend your time.

It is important that you take the time to recall and establish who you are so that you can begin to develop your identity outside of the addiction. Codependence gets us so wrapped up in the anxiety of the loved one's addic-tion that we lose ourselves in the process. Committing to doing these activities can get you started on rekindling a strong sense of yourself. Try to discover the things that you love or even the activities you aren't very interested in because those are some of the building blocks to honoring what you need in order to experience the fullness of your life. Unfortunately, aside from accountability, there is nothing you can do to force the ad-dict to stop damaging his life—but you do not have to lose your life in the process as well.

CHAPTER 8

Nurturing Your Soul: Uncovering Your Zest for Life

__Meditation for Today:__ Our life light is bright, and struggles can dim it with chaos and worries. Consider: what lights you up and energizes you? What parts of life bring you joy or fill you with the sweetness of bliss and contentment? Take a moment and allow those images and feelings to surge through your body, letting the warmth of pleasant feelings consume you, even for this one moment today.

Do you know or remember the things that make you feel a zest for living? Zest for life is about tapping into the spirit of truly living your life awake, instead of just getting by, going through the motions, and hoping you can sleep through the night. A person who is going through the motions is simply surviving. Think of this as being in survival mode. This is a kind of living that keeps you from seeing the vibrancy and beauty that still exist in the world—the true colors that have been overshadowed for so long by your worries and fears about your loved one.

Finding enthusiasm for your life is possible. As you do this, some of the worry thoughts may enter your mind: Am I being selfish? Shouldn't I be doing something? How can I enjoy my life while my loved one is suffering? Be aware: these are simply thoughts. You don't have to buy into them or believe them. They will undoubtedly rise up in your mind, especially if you are truly (re)discovering yourself and your zest for your life. These thoughts may try to trick you into going back to just surviving because that is what you know, or what feels most comfortable. But the challenge will be to take a leap of faith and get out of your comfort zone. In doing this, you will be overcoming the addiction in your own life, and *you* will not be letting the addiction win.

Addiction is a family dis-ease. It impacts everyone in different ways and leaves everyone in the family system with different types of pain and hurt. You will have to overcome this in your own life, and in doing so, you will prove that addiction can truly be beaten. However, it will take focusing and refocusing on your priorities. If your life becomes consumed by the priority of the addiction (i.e., going back to war with it and letting it control your life), then you will also be falling back into dis-ease. Remember: the only element of your life that you can truly change is yourself. If you have been consumed with the worries and obsessions about your loved one, then you have also been feeding the addiction. In taking back your life and truly living it with joy, compassion, and empathy, you will relinquish the hold the dis-ease has over you. You will have more truly authentic compassion, love, and resources to provide your loved ones when or if they decide to enter into the same spirit of recovery.

Think of this process as getting back to the basics of your life—if you can remember what that was like! If not, it's time to figure out what drives you. What inspires and compels you into joy and a zest for living? Some of this you have likely discovered in previous chapters. After the previous Survival Steps, you have hopefully started acting on some of these to take care of yourself in the most basic ways (food, exercise, and mental health) and can now enter into more robust living.

Survival Step: Name this state of living for yourself—the one where you are finding your zest for life, rather than just surviving and getting by. In doing so, you will create a mantra, or a reminder, of what your daily goal is.

- Name it: "[your name] Basics"—I always use my nickname—"Reesa Basics," but use whatever form of your name that will remind you that you are getting back to the basics of living with joy and excitement.

  ____

- Now, come up with a reminder phrase that is easy to remember, using the name you gave this style of living—"I need to get back to Reesa Basics." This will be important to remember when you are starting to feel overwhelmed or stressed, as it will cue you to get refocused on your priorities. Write your short reminder phrase here: _______________________________

  ____.

Remember, you aren't doing anything wrong if you start to feel overwhelmed or stressed. Of course you feel this way! Life certainly has its fair share of stress and heartache, plus you are struggling to accept and manage the emotional impacts of someone you love hurting themselves or others with addiction. These emotions will come and go, and it will be important that you have a quick way to remind yourself to get back to the basics of truly living—fulfilled and joyfully.

CHAPTER 9

Securing Serenity: Calm in the Chaos of Addiction

__Meditation for Today:__ Take a moment to scan your body, from head to toe. Focus on trying to relax any parts of your body that may carry tension or stress. Use your breath to direct energy and focus to any places that need to give you ease and calm. Touch serenity by softening your body and quieting the thoughts in your mind.

You have done a lot of work on who you are and where you are in your journey. You have reviewed information on addiction, its impacts, and your role in healing yourself from the dis-ease in your life. Moving forward, one of the most important things to remember is that all of this is an ongoing process. It is important to be gentle with yourself and others because there will be moments you wish you had chosen a different direction or different words, and you may feel angry when others make decisions that hurt you and their own lives. There will be times you will find yourself dipping back into despair about the addiction and its impact on you or your family members' lives, but it is important that you don't get stuck in the despair.

Acceptance is the most important, crucial part of Security Serenity. There are several aspects of acceptance that are important to consider. To "accept," according to the *Merriam-Webster Dictionary*, is "to receive willingly." To think about acceptance is to consider the act of receiving willingly. Or rather, not resisting willfully. Acceptance is necessary for moving forward in the journey of healing, and it is not something we can do just once and consider it complete. While discovering more about this concept, think of "acceptance" as a verb, or an action word, rather than a noun, or a thing. It is something that requires energy and action from the person trying to find it. Through actively accepting and receiving willingly, you will begin to secure and deepen your serenity.

It is difficult to imagine accepting something that feels so stressful or devastating. When you love someone who is struggling with addiction, your first reaction very likely may be to reject acceptance. You may think,

"*No way* am I going to accept what my loved one is doing to ruin her life! I can't be okay with that; I have to do something!" However, even when examining the meaning of that thought, it is clear that the person thinking it is spending a lot of energy rejecting reality. Of course you will think like this sometimes, but having these beliefs certainly doesn't help the addict, and it will only make you suffer more. So what does it mean to take an active stance on acceptance?

First, it is important to know that acceptance is not to be confused with *permission* or *consent*. These concepts are very different from acceptance. Many times, though, when we are not okay with something (i.e., not consenting to it), we fight it. When you love someone who is struggling with addiction, you are not going to be okay with that person's behavior. However, can you change their behavior? No. Absolutely not. You can change your responses to the person's behavior, but you cannot change the addict. When we move into acceptance, this means we are living in the moment and not fighting reality. Fighting what *is* takes significant time and energy away from us and leaves us feeling helpless and ineffective because when it comes down to it, we cannot change another person. We can only move into a place of acceptance and peace within our own lives.

Just as acceptance isn't giving consent or permission for something, it also doesn't mean sitting idly by and allowing the dis-ease to run rampant in your life. When you accept what is true at this very moment, it empowers you to decide how you want to respond, rather than living in a manner that fights reality and makes you feel exhausted. Fighting reality looks different for everyone who is living with addiction, but there are some common themes: agonizing over the decisions your loved one is making to the point that it is interfering with other activities, sleep, or overall health; spending time hounding and berating the addict about his or her choices; living with frequent battles and tension; or living in denial of the person's behavior, making excuses for what they do and supporting the addiction through your own behaviors. All of these things can be signs that you are fighting what *is*, and your fight will only lead you deeper into a life of chaos and misery.

Acceptance is the key tool that brings everything together in the quest of securing serenity. Serenity is akin to peace, but it is so much more. It is finding the center of peace and wisdom inside yourself, even in the biggest storm. Serenity can be described by imagining an incredibly still, peaceful body of water. When a pebble is thrown into it, what happens to the water? The pebble will create ripples, yes, but the pond does not work and strain to toss the pebble back out. It does not fight and groan or dry up and disappear. It accepts and accommodates and returns to its original state without much fuss. We want to strive to be like this. As human beings, the goal is not to be unaffected by the difficulties we encounter, but rather, to honor and accept the difficulties and discern when action must be taken. Eastern philosophy uses a metaphor of running water in a stream. When the water encounters any kind of branch, rock, or barrier, the running water doesn't fight or resist the barrier. It doesn't halt its forward movement and insist that the rock move. It simply parts and flows around it, going along to its next destination. Such is the way that we need to be with problems that we cannot change. Give in to the flow of life, without letting it wash you away.

Acceptance isn't easy, and it isn't a onetime-fits-forever decision. Know that when you move into a spirit of acceptance, you are not lying down and saying it is okay. You can still decide how you want to respond, and you *must* do so. It is important to carefully consider the wisdom in your response and choose what is going to move you along toward success and well-being. Do not waste time on fruitless efforts to force others to change. Accept what is, in this very moment, and try not to focus all your energy on what has happened, or may happen in the future. Accept and live in this moment, securing your serenity in order to live your life joyfully and with abundance.

Survival Step: Take two to three minutes to consider the areas in your life where you continue to resist and fight the addiction. As you try to find these, think about the areas that stress you out, or times when your thoughts reject reality. Now jot down some of the ideas you have.

____

____

____

Survival Step: Write a letter to yourself in which you give yourself permission to move into a state of acceptance related to the addiction in your life. Consider how you can let go of the relentless internal and external fight against the reality of the circumstances.

____

____

____

____

____

____

Survival Step: Now find someone you trust, and ask them to sit with you while you read the letter out loud to him or her. Ask this person to help you remember your commitment to acceptance. As the Serenity Prayer points out, you have to keep reminding yourself of your commitment to accept what you cannot change while continuing to change what you can—and when we share our commitments with others, we are more likely to be successful in keeping them.

Survival Step: Read and familiarize yourself with the Serenity Prayer. It is a helpful mantra to re-center yourself on your priority of acceptance.

Grant me the serenity to
Accept the things I cannot change,
Courage to change the things I can,
And wisdom to know the difference.
-Reinhold Niebuhr

Remember: "Serenity is not freedom from the storm, but peace amid the storm" -Anonymous

CHAPTER 10

Investing in Spirituality: What It Means for Your Journey

__Meditation for Today:__ Hope never hurts. Take a moment to pause and consider that short phrase. Let it settle down inside of your mind and your heart and consider how you can develop a relationship with Hope while releasing any illusion of control over the addiction.

n thinking of spirituality here, try to broaden your understanding of what that word represents. Spirituality goes far beyond what we usually think of: religion, doctrine, and prayer. In the context of recovery, consider spirituality as a concept of looking for the source of your serenity—your peace of spirit. It is a personal practice for your soul that leads you to a strong sense of purpose, destiny, well-being, and connection with the world around you. Religious studies can certainly be a tool in nurturing your spirituality, but as we all know, the connection of the words and ideas come at a deeply spiritual level.

One tool that is extremely helpful in discovering and deepening your spirituality is mindfulness. Mindfulness is applied in many Eastern religions, but you will also find elements of it steeped in many Western practices. It isn't exclusive to any one religion or practice. You don't have to aspire to be a Buddhist monk or a Yogi to practice and master your ability to be mindful. Christians also practice mindfulness in prayer and gratitude, among other areas. It can become a part of your daily life in some very easy steps.

What is mindfulness? It is having the ability to be connected with *this moment* and all the fullness and opportunity it offers. You may be sitting there doing this workbook and thinking that this moment is just an ordinary one. But it isn't. Not just because you are working on something that will profoundly affect your life, but because there is richness and vitality in every moment that frequently goes unnoticed or unnamed. Look around you right now. Notice all of your senses, and connect them with the present moment. Breathe in *all* that this moment can offer to you.

Why practice mindfulness? When we are connected in the here and now, it allows us to have more mastery over our emotions and thoughts. We are no longer idle passengers to thoughts, judgments, perceptions, and beliefs that may not serve us well. So many times, it is the reality our brains create that keeps us from experiencing the joy or serenity of the moment. These also allow the worries, fears, and anxieties about parts of our lives, which are not in front of us right now, to get in the way of truly being connected with our current circumstances. Thus, we often miss out on our own lives. Really, as much as it is a cliché, all we are truly guaranteed is this very moment. When you can exercise your ability to connect and live fully in this moment, the richness of your life and spirituality increases exponentially.

How do we do mindfulness? It can be incorporated into every moment of your life. You can take a moment to be connected right now. You can appreciate and revel in some of the smallest routines in your life and find value in them. One important part of mindfulness is increasing and improving your ability to notice when your mind has judgmental thoughts and recognizing that these are just thoughts. Thoughts and our judgments about the world around us are not necessarily an accurate representation of what is truly around us. By recognizing and increasing awareness of your internal judgments and dialogue, you will improve your ability to master your emotions. Just because you *think it* doesn't necessarily make it absolute truth. We all have judgments, and there is nothing wrong with having them. Your task will be to improve your ability to discern which judgments are helpful to you and which ones create more pain or suffering. If they do not help you and/or are not true, then the thoughts don't serve you well. As you are aware of how your brain interprets the environment, you will be able to truly hone in on the truth and power of now and *decide* how you want to think or feel about the moment.

Survival Step: The most easily accessible way to settle into mindfulness is to connect with your senses. So take a moment and go through all of your senses and just notice what you observe. If your brain has any judgments or gets distracted, just pull your mind back to the moment through your senses.

Now write down to describe, without judgmental words, what your senses observed—try to even stay away from words like "good" or "fun" or "bad" and just describe what you noticed:

____

____

____

____

____

Write down any judgments you noticed as you were doing the mindfulness practice:

____

____

____

____

____

Notice what your judgments may add or subtract from the current moment. Now decide what is true for *you*. What do you want to believe? For example, as I tune into my sense of touch right now, I notice that my back is touching the chair. Then I notice, "Ouch, my back is sore. I shouldn't have slept wrong last night." If I continue to let my thoughts focus on something painful in the moment, it subtracts from my joy right now. So I have a decision to make, and I can choose to shift my attention back to this moment. I do this by placing my focus on my breathing and relaxing my body. I notice the feeling of the chair on my back and the support it gives. Yes, I can also notice for a moment that my back is sore. But I am not going to let my thoughts continue into other judgmental territory about "should have, could have, would have," or let my mind continue to focus on pain. I will move on to another part of the experience right now and remember to take care of my back as I move forward.

As you live your life each day, you can choose where your mind spends its time. When it encounters each moment, your brain and thoughts may be conditioned to respond in a certain way. Increasing your awareness of your judgments will allow you to alter those experiences in any way you want. If you want to have more positive thoughts, then you have the power to do so. If you want something to change, instead of sitting with suffering, judgments, and recriminations, you have the power to go out and change it. Or, in most cases, you can simply invest yourself fully in this moment and experience the abundance it has to offer, instead of living in the past or worrying about an uncertain future.

Survival Step: Think of a task you have done today that is a part of your daily routine. Something you do almost without thinking. For example, "I am going to reflect mindfully on making and drinking my cup of coffee this morning. I can observe this experience and find gratitude for so many elements of this task. I am grateful for the hands to make the coffee, the grounds that are created, the store I bought it from, the smell of the roast as it brews," and so on. Select a daily activity and really observe and describe it in detail:

Activity: _______________________________
What do you observe about this that you rarely notice?

____

____

____

____

____

____

Survival Step: Each day, tune in to at least one moment and practice this heightened awareness of your senses and observations. Track your experiences throughout the week. Allow yourself to truly experience the activity each day with 100 percent of yourself. Create a reminder somewhere—maybe an alarm in your phone, a Post-it note, or something else that will help you to remember to notice that moment and observe all of your senses or your breathing. The more you make time to practice this, the more you will notice mastery over your experiences and fully live in the present moment. You will begin to understand the power you have over where you focus your thoughts and attention.

Day	What senses you notice	Observations about the experience

Day	What senses you notice	Observations about the experience

Survival Step: Notice your breathing. Even more than your senses, the in and out of your breath is something you will *always* have access to. It will never leave you, so long as you are still alive. It is the only thing that is your constant companion, and you can control and influence it. Your breathing also helps to fuel your body and brain. When your brain has the oxygen it needs, you can think more clearly and make better decisions to take care of yourself and your environment. So use this tool at any time because it is always there.

- In this moment, breathe in and out slowly and steadily three times. Inhale through your nose deeply and slowly, and then exhale through your mouth until you have pushed out all the air you can. Tune in to the experience.

- When your mind is particularly full of distracting or worrisome thoughts, it can be helpful to pick out one or two words that you repeat on the inhale and exhale. For example, breathe in the word "peace," and exhale "now." Do this three or four times—use your own words/phrases that guide you toward what you need in the moment. Allow it to clear your mind and focus your attention on this moment.

In sum, you have the power to change your perception of the world, and it starts with using the tools you have to be mindful of and connect with the wholeness of your spirit. Find connection to the life that surrounds you in a meaningful, deep way. By adopting these practices, you will deepen your spirituality and find the essence of truly living your life with abundance.

CHAPTER 11

Long-Term Recovery of the Spirit That Lasts: Permanent Change for You

__Meditation for Today:__ Consider these wise words and their implications for your journey: "All changes, even the most longed for, have their melancholy; for what we leave behind us is a part of ourselves. We must die to one life before we can enter another." -Anatole France

Sometimes it feels selfish to move forward with your life. And sometimes it will be lonely and scary to venture into this new world in which you have left the obsession about the loved one's addiction behind. But you have done so much work to have gotten this far. Review this workbook when you feel the pull of the dis-ease trying to get you back into its clutches. Just because someone in your life is living with addiction doesn't mean you have to be controlled by it too. In fact, if a loved one is living with addiction, you owe it to yourself and to your family members to first break its hold on you, and then live the life you want. By doing this, you can be a living example of someone moving out of the vise-grip of addiction and into a life of recovery. Then don't forget to pray and hope that your loved one also finds his or her peace of spirit and mind.

Moving forward into this new way of living allows you to love deeply and with the full commitment of your spirit. You will be released from the chains of addiction that bind you, too, and you can be a living example of healing. Then you will be able to be there for your family and loved ones in a different way. If you decide that you must make some life-changing decisions in this process, such as ending a relationship because it is causing suffering, you will find the strength and courage within yourself to live, love, and laugh as you move forward in your life. It will be very hard but also necessary. Only you know the true wisdom and answers within yourself. When you have done the work to remove the dis-ease's hold on your life, you remove the chaos that keeps your soul from knowing its own wisdom. With that chaos in place, it keeps us from loving ourselves and others the way we want to—the way we know brings fulfillment and harmony into our lives.

This workbook was never designed to *give* you the answers, but rather to guide you to your own wisdom and truth. If there is one thing that loving someone with an addiction has taught me, it's that all of life is about living "in the gray." Very few situations fit into the black-and-white categories of good or bad and right or wrong. Truth is always somewhere in the middle. It's in the gray area where the real work is done and love can grow and change you from the inside out. Whatever you decide to do, look deep within after having completed the work in this book and see what comes next. For some, it may be ending a hard relationship. For others, it may be seeking out therapy and personal support through community meetings. There is so much love and support out there. If you feel like you are alone, you don't have to be. Find the services and relationships that are out there waiting for you. This workbook is not going to be the only tool you will need in your journey of keeping addiction from holding on to the reins of control in your life. Many others out there share in parts of your journey and in seeking to find the truth and healing that is within each of us.

The final thoughts as we move ahead in our personal journeys of recovery are to seek to live passionately because this moment and this life are all we are guaranteed. It is important to keep working on your attitude by using the mindfulness tools to help keep your mindset the way you want it to be. Continue seeking wisdom and acceptance from these experiences. Be willing to take chances and love as many people and things as you can each day. The beauty of love is that there is no limit to the amount we all have to give to others. So love on.

Find ways to celebrate your life and successes, even in the smallest ways—such as starting a gratitude journal to give celebration and thanks for even the smallest things you may have ordinarily missed. Tune in to your senses at different times during each day to truly celebrate and honor the moment. Find pleasure in the smallest things, and experience them at maximum capacity. Wake up each day with the mindset of choosing an attitude of investing in yourself and in your peace of mind. When challenges arise, I often remind myself to "be like water," meaning to go with the flow. I know I learned this from stories about wisdom and flexibility—something that, as a recovering dis-eased person, was really tough for me. I wanted to control and change things and other people and push them to bend to my will, but that never lead to anything other than more suffering.

Live today. Live now. Work to make sure that you are keeping as much energy invested in yourself and your well-being as you do for others. You cannot truly be there for and love people the way your heart desires without starting with yourself. Thank you for taking this journey with me. I am truly honored to have been a part of your healing and I hope that you have found wisdom and inspiration in your hard work. You are amazing, strong, and resilient and have everything you need to live the life you have always wanted.

For one final **Survival Step** to close out our work together, consider this question: What is next for me in living life free of dis-ease and full of love, compassion, and serenity?

Helpful Resources:

- Al-Anon: 12-step support meetings for family and friends who have been impacted by a loved one's substance addiction: www.al-anon.org
- Nar-anon: 12-step support meetings for family and friends who have been impacted by a loved one's substance addiction: www.nar-anon.org
- Gam-anon: 12-step support groups for family and friends who have been impacted by a loved one's gambling addiction: www.gam-anon.org
- CoDA: Codependents Anonymous International, for people seeking to develop healthy relationships: CoDA.org
- Adult Children of Alcoholics World Service Organization: a community for adult children of alcoholics and addicts: www.adultchildren.org
- Partnership for Drug-Free Kids: resources for parents and caregivers of a youth struggling with addiction (includes a parent blog): drugfree.org
- Substance Abuse and Mental Health Services Administration (SAMHSA): www.samhsa.gov
- Book: *Beautiful Boy: A Father's Journey Through His Son's Addiction* by David Sheff
- Book: *Codependent No More* by Melody Beattie
- Book: *The Power of Now: A Guide to Spiritual Enlightenment* by Eckhart Tolle
- Online articles, books, and videos (many of them free) to teach more about mindfulness
- Mindfulness and meditation practice: browse free or low-cost applications available for download on smartphones
- Contact your local community mental health center for therapy, support, and guidance on other resources available in your neighborhood